Beginning an ACADEMIC MEDICAL CAREER

Research, Writing, Speaking

Reginald C. Tsang, M.B.B.S.
and
William Oh, M.D.
with the assistance of
Lynda L. Price, R.N., M.A.

Publisher: Digital Educational Publishing, Inc.
P.O. Box 43515
Cincinnati, OH 45243

BEGINNING AN ACADEMIC
MEDICAL CAREER ISBN 978-1-56053-064-0

Library of Congress catalog card number 92-74264

Last digit is the print number: 9 8 7 6 5 4 3 2 1

About the Authors

Reginald C. Tsang, M.B.B.S., is Gamble Professor of Neonatology, and Professor of Pediatrics and Obstetrics at the University of Cincinnati College of Medicine and Children's Hospital Medical Center, Cincinnati, Ohio. As Director of the Perinatal Research Institute, he has been involved in training young academicians for two decades and brings his knowledge and experience to this subject in an interesting and often humorous way. Dr. Tsang's research interests are calcium and nutrition. He is the author of *Vitamin and Mineral Requirements in Preterm Infants* and *Nutrition During Infancy*, two acclaimed reference texts for nutrition in infancy. He is the Principal Investigator of the NIH Diabetes in Pregnancy Program Project and the Perinatal Emphasis Research Center at the University of Cincinnati and Children's Hospital.

William Oh, M.D., is Professor and Chairman, Department of Pediatrics at Brown University Program in Medicine, and Pediatrician-in-Chief at the Women and Infants Hospital and Rhode Island Hospital, Providence, Rhode Island. Dr. Oh is the Principal Investigator of the Rhode Island Perinatal Emphasis Research Center. As an experienced scientist in perinatal medicine, he contributes his administrative and research experience to this important aspect of an academic career.

Lynda L. Price, R.N., M.A., is Director of Human Resources, University of Cincinnati Medical Center, Cincinnati, Ohio. She combines a medical background with several years of experience in teaching professional writing to create publications for medical and nonmedical readers.

Acknowledgments

The authors gratefully acknowledge the help of a number of individuals in an earlier version of this book as well as the current text: William Balistreri, M.D., Cincinnati, OH; Jeffrey Maisels, MBBS, Detroit, MI; Dewey Sehring, Ross Laboratories, Columbus, OH; Robert Merrill, M.D., Philadelphia, PA; and Stan Ward, Philadelphia, PA.

Distribution of this book is made possible, in part, by Ross Laboratories, Columbus, Ohio.

We extend special thanks to Brian Epp and Regina Hasson for the illustrations.

Contents

The greatest use of a life is to spend it for something that will outlast it.

William James

Introduction

To start a career in academic medicine is exciting, but there are many pitfalls and frustrations. To write a paper is exciting, but many have trouble getting the first sentence on paper. To write a grant application is also exciting, but can be frustrating. We like to remind our fellows that while it may be difficult to write a grant application, "One thing is certain, if you never write a grant application, you will never get a grant." To give a talk can be exciting, and may even be inspiring to some members of your audience; but you can also be an absolute bore and lose every listener.

This book is intended to help you start an exciting career that should never be dull.

> *Writing is an adventure. To begin with, it is a toy and an amusement. Then it becomes a mistress, then it becomes a master, then it becomes a tyrant. The last phase is that just as you are about to be reconciled to your servitude, you kill the monster and fling him to the public.*
>
> Sir Winston Churchill (1932)

Foreword

This small book by renowned professors Reggie Tsang and William Oh should be considered required reading for all young academics beginning their careers in medicine, and is strongly recommended to faculty who serve as mentors. First published about twenty years ago, the crisp and sagacious guidance provided in this book remains true and on target. Each previous publication of the book has been "sold out" with copies passed from person to person, and used to guide faculty careers in academic medical centers throughout the U.S. and internationally. We expect that this re-publication will be just as popular.

Getting started in academic medicine is a daunting process. Where does one begin? The book begins with how to get started on your own project, including how to find problems worthy of sustained attention; how to find effective mentors and create professional networks; the importance of "focus, focus, focus" to develop depth of expertise and true innovation in the defined arena; and how to set yourself apart from others in your field. The book does not provide a short-cut to hard work and self-discipline, but rather provides the committed young academic with the advice needed to use their time and effort effectively, whether strategizing about their career development, presenting a talk, writing a manuscript, developing an hypothesis, writing a grant application, preparing a curriculum vitae, or developing the ability to think critically. The advice is direct and practical, infused with a positive outlook that makes the reader confident that, "I can do this!"

Cincinnati Children's Hospital Medical Center has an unwavering commitment to the development of its trainees and junior faculty, who are clearly the future of this institution and of pediatrics. As part of that commitment, Cincinnati Children's Research Foundation has supported publication of this book to make it again available to this generation of young academics who need this career development guidance as much as ever.

Thomas F. Boat, MD
Chairman, Department of Pediatrics,
University of Cincinnati College of Medicine
B.K. Rachford Professor of Pediatrics
Director, Cincinnati Children's Research Foundation

This book, first provided to me in 1990 by my mentor, has been my "career bible" ever since. I have derived encouragement and practical guidance from it, shared and given away countless copies, and quoted from it as I became a mentor and lecturer. Only later did I meet Reggie Tsang and correspond with William Oh, and put the life story together with the text of the book. The long and the short of it – these professors have lived and taught what they wrote, and exemplify the successful academic life and how to live it with good humor. The smart young academic will treasure the pearls in this book and use them wisely.

Ardythe L. Morrow, PhD
Professor of Pediatrics
University of Cincinnati College of Medicine
Director, Center for Epidemiology and Biostatistics
Cincinnati Children's Hospital Medical Center

Chapter 1

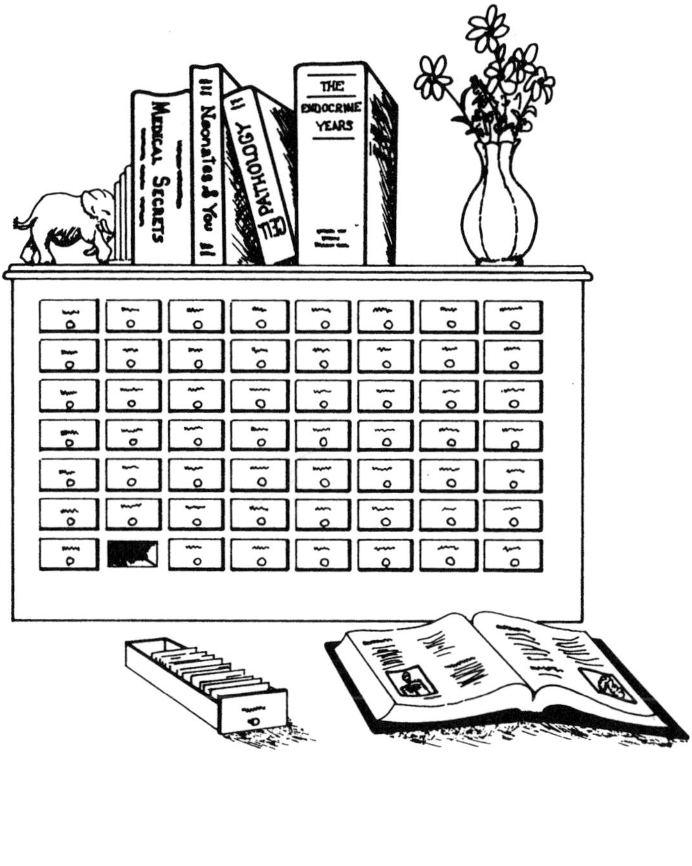

Developing Your Project and Designing Your Study

1

Developing Your Project and Designing Your Study

And, as imagination bodies forth
The forms of things unknown, the poet's pen
Turns them into shapes, and gives to airy nothing
A focal habitation and a name.

William Shakespeare
Midsummer Night's Dream V.i.14–17

One of the most important first steps in an academic career is to develop your own project. While the project is still in your imagination, seek out the best people in your environment. Pick their brains! Barrage them with questions and use them as sounding boards for your ideas. Let them help map out the global view. They can point you toward the major gaps of understanding in your field. Interacting with the experts will help to determine the feasibility of your ideas and to formulate the exact focus of your project.

Set yourself apart. Find an area of interest that has not been previously explored or has been explored minimally. Sometimes, exploring areas that were touched on a long time ago, when techniques and methods were relatively "primitive," works well. You want an area in which you can be identified for the next five to ten years.

In finding this niche, you should determine that the project will eventually lead to results that are clinically or biologically relevant—or both. The results should point toward new areas for investigation. In other words, select an area that will continue to open new vistas over the years. Map out the plan by a series of logical steps, including "what if" steps, to help forecast the possible course of events. Also make sure the project is possible from the standpoint of both available techniques and design.

Many young academic physicians believe that in a few years they will exhaust the subject they set out to explore and that they will need to study another subject. This is rarely the case. Your distinguished senior professors are not working on the same problems with which they began, but they can trace their current interests thirty or forty years to their initial investigations. If you have the opportunity, examine the curriculum vitae of some distinguished senior professors.

In determining your area of interest, remember that a narrow focus results in a deep and sophisticated understanding of the subject, which then allows you to progress logically to the next (albeit unseen) steps. A broad focus, however, locks you into a superficial treatment of a subject and limits the ability to generate new ideas because you are not expert enough to move beyond a merely interesting initial observation. If you begin with a narrow focus and add the inevitable improvement in research skills, your interests will automatically broaden. But wherever your narrowly focused interests eventually lead, you must resist the common temptation to cover too wide a field.

Remember your major interest and whittle away at that topic until you reach a narrow focus. It is much more interesting to climb the only peak that has never been climbed than to be the fiftieth person to climb Mt. Kilimanjaro.

> *You should do research because you enjoy it, not because you want to be immortalized.*
>
> Helen Harrison, Ph.D.
> Johns Hopkins
> Baltimore, Maryland

Select your preceptors carefully. If you select a junior preceptor, always find a senior preceptor as well, so that both can be apprised of your progress throughout your training. Constantly feed them information so that they can understand your interests and will be able to interact intelligently with you. They are your sounding board, your conscience, your critics, and your sources of encouragement; hence they must be well informed about your area of interest. Your goal should be to develop knowledge and expertise so that you exceed the knowledge of all your preceptors. Thus, you must identify and follow a unique course. You must establish yourself as the independent investigator. *You* become the expert.

> *Work with a person you admire.*
>
> Frank Oski, M.D.
> Johns Hopkins
> Baltimore, Maryland

Develop your critical abilities. After choosing your topic, read every piece of literature on the topic. Dissect all previous studies thoroughly, incisively, and critically. Identify their weaknesses. Avoid a study simply to improve a previous study slightly; rather, assess the major gaps in knowledge and set out to fill them.

> *It is a sad student who cannot exceed his preceptor.*
>
> William Balistreri, M.D.
> Children's Hospital
> Cincinnati, Ohio

Devise a plan. Having found a topic, sit down and map out short- and long-term plans. What can you honestly accomplish in two or three years? What can be achieved with the resources and expertise available? What is not available?

Both short- and long-range plans will help in your overall career development. Your short-term plans will help focus your research activity and maximize productivity during your fellowship years. These in turn provide the basis for your next academic appointment. The long-term plan helps to keep career goals in focus and enhances the ability to choose the best institution in which to continue your research.

Remember that nothing is more critical in the research proposal than the hypothesis. Define your hypothesis clearly. Do not make statements such as, "We will observe the changes. . . ." That is not a hypothesis; it is a general statement. Instead, state your hypothesis ***specifically:*** "An increase in A will result in a decrease in B." Not only have you identified the specific subject and object, you have also defined the ***direction*** of change. You have put yourself out on a limb by defining your expectations. This clear and specifically stated hypothesis will force you to defend the pros and cons of your position thoroughly in your text.

Have the hypothesis in front of you as you write the proposal. The ***introduction*** should emphasize the pros and cons of your position and the hypothetical reasons for any putative changes. For example, after synthesizing the available literature, your hunch may be that the change should be an increase. Work with that assumption throughout your proposal. As you present your ***plan and methods,*** choose those that allow you to evaluate whether increases or decreases in measurements are present. But merely ascertaining which is not enough; the implications must be examined. If there is an increase, is there a response that is in the "toxic" range, particularly for human subjects? In this case you need to resolve the problem of toxicity. If there is a decrease, will there be a "deficiency" condition? You need to describe the precautions you plan to undertake to minimize potentially adverse effects. ***Thus, your clearly stated hypothesis sets the stage for utilizing precise methods that can appropriately assess the changes in measures.***

Read about and attend courses on biostatistics and study design. Some excellent references on biostatistics and study design are listed in the section "Recommended Reading." Research involves unending study of these areas. Somewhere in your institution you can find a biostatistics group. Make contact with them, acquaint them with your areas of interest, and attend their lectures; they will be your lifelong friends and collaborators.

Avoid "fishing" expeditions. They have little place in science. If twenty things are measured, one is likely to be significant by definition. Science involves focus; test only one or two things at a time. Always ask yourself whether this is a fishing expedition or a real hypothesis. Fishing often kills your abstract or paper and will always kill your grant.

Evaluate outside resources. Be aware of the best resources and expertise available. If necessary, visit another department in your institution, or another medical center, to be in touch with the best minds and methods. The methods of your research are critical; learn them thoroughly and well, from every available source. Control of your methods is what makes you and your science special.

Ensure a system in which quality is maintained throughout. What is the ***gold standard*** and does the gold standard change? How often is the assay checked against the gold standard? What is the coefficient of variation of the assay? Who will perform the assay? One technician? Two? Three? Reduce the number of technicians to the absolute minimum to reduce potential problems.

Perform all the major assays yourself. There is only one way to understand the rationale of an assay or its methods as well as how to "trouble-shoot" it, and that is to do it yourself. Dr. Jeff Maisels, who reviewed this book in manuscript, states, "I used to run my carbon monoxide assays between 11 p.m. and 4 a.m., after completing a study, because the elevators didn't run much at those hours. The elevators affected the line voltage on our 'Model T' gas chromatograph."

Never do during the day what you can do at night.

Frank Oski, M.D.
Johns Hopkins
Baltimore, Maryland

Plan to run all assays (or other similar measurements) in one batch, if possible. This will minimize interassay variability.

Ensure that samples do not deteriorate in storage. Determine how long samples can be stored and what storage precautions must be taken.

I hear and I forget
I see and I remember
I do and I understand.

Old Chinese Proverb

This is why you must **do** *research, just as you must perform clinical skills.*

William W. Hay, Jr., M.D.
University of Colorado
Health Sciences Center
Denver, Colorado

Have a thorough grasp of quality-control aspects of assays performed in other laboratories, if you work outside your department or institution. Go over all steps of each procedure with personnel from the other laboratory. Observe each step from beginning to end, from sample collection to data output. Each step is vital, and deviation could mean disaster for your project.

Consult with your preceptor frequently as you plan your strategy. Both of you should evaluate the merits and demerits of your plan.

Discovery consists of seeing what everyone else has seen but thinking what no one else has thought.

Albert Gyorgy

Locate at least three or four highly qualified and highly critical reviewers who will review your written study proposal.

Arrange one or two meetings at which the early drafts of your proposal are presented formally. Reviewers and others need to evaluate your ideas critically. Encourage hypercritical reactions during the early stage of the proposal. It is much better to accept criticism at this stage of the project, and much easier to revise your strategy, than to work for three years and then discover that you overlooked an important aspect.

Develop a strong support system. Cultivate friends and colleagues in addition to your preceptors. This group will become your true friends who will support, criticize, and encourage you. They will function as catalysts for your continued intellectual stimulation and as mentors for successful research. Select them carefully and remain loyal to them. Keep them posted and send updates and reprints to keep them abreast of your field, at least in the major areas of your research. This information will enable your reviewers to criticize and interact with you intelligently.

> *Real success in academic medicine requires a mentor, an important project, perseverence, and patience. Fame does not come overnight. As an unidentified sage has stated: 'All things cometh to him who waiteth if he worketh like hell while he waiteth.'*
>
> Delbert A. Fisher, M.D.
> Harbor-UCLA Medical Center
> Torrance, California

Join journal club discussions. Use this chapter and Chapter 7 as a checklist: Is there a hypothesis? Is there a clear study description?

Reviewing papers with a group provides a lively way of improving your ability to read a paper, as the discussion will be tempered by the biases that surface in any group interaction. Remember to keep an objective mind, and try to distinguish between objective and subjective comments. Volunteer to assist your mentor in reviewing articles sent from reputable journals for critiques. As you work with your mentor, you will hone your own analytic skills and improve your instincts for appropriate study design.

> *The most important requirement for an academician is an incredible sense of humor.*
>
> Harry L. Greene, M.D.
> Vanderbilt University
> Nashville, Tennessee

Realize that if you have written the study proposal and hypotheses clearly, all the points will flow smoothly when you write the manuscript. For example, you should have introduced the rationale and hypothesis for why a particular finding is expected. You hypothesize that the hormone concentration should go up; if you find that the hormone level did rise, discuss why the data are consistent with the original hypothesis. If the results show the opposite, it is even more important to attempt a reconciliation. It may be that these diametrically opposite results are "the beginning of a new symphony." You may have discovered something startling, and in that case you will be able to pursue a new line of reasoning contrary to previous knowledge. By hypothesizing a specific direction of change, you have locked yourself into a system of debate that provokes clear thought and presentation.

> *Reading maketh a full man; conference a ready man; and writing an exact man.*
>
> Sir Francis Bacon (1588)

Chapter 2

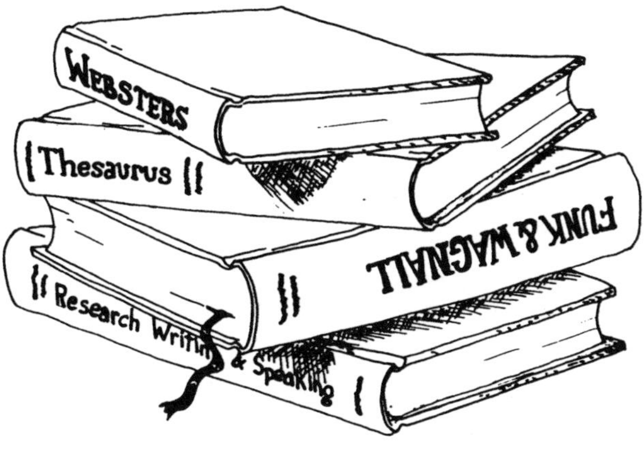

Writing Abstracts for Scientific Meeting Presentations

2

Writing Abstracts for Scientific Meeting Presentations

Handle them carefully, for words have more power than atom bombs.

Pearl Strachan Hurd (1935)

Abstract writing is one of those arts that you must learn quickly and well. All of your professional presentations will be accepted or rejected on the basis of how well you write the abstract, so approach this task with a clear and precise mind. ***Every word counts.*** Committee members who review abstracts usually have many responsibilities and other distractions. They also receive many abstracts; therefore, yours needs to stand out. Be sharp! "Many are culled, but few are chosen."

Keep the title simple, factual, and interesting. Relate the title to your hypothesis. Attract your readers' attention. Boldly state your position. Avoid irrelevance. Be selective.

Keep the introduction simple. State ***why*** you did the study. Write direct sentences. Whet your readers' appetites to learn more about the project by highlighting the issue of concern. Be as specific as possible.

Keep in mind that the hypothesis is the most important part of the abstract. State it clearly. If you state your hypothesis precisely and specifically, you have sharpened the abstract immeasurably.

Distinguish yourself by identifying a new procedure or a new point of view in the Methods section. Whatever is new has some value (although it might not be immediately useful). Highlight the parts you think are most interesting and minimize the rest. It becomes a matter of balance.

Remember that the bulk of the abstract is contained in the Results section. Pack it with precise data. Give exact values; for example, mean ± standard error. Focus on a few of the more interesting points. Put your best and most relevant data early in the text to attract readers' attention. Put your best foot forward! Be precise about which statistical tests were performed and on ***which data.***

Avoid abbreviations or acronyms that are not standard. Spell out an abbreviation or acronym the first time it appears in the text.

Write a strong conclusion. After reading the abstract, the reviewer should be confident that you have adequately tested your hypothesis, have data to support it, and have concluded the project. Many abstracts contain a conclusion that is speculative rather than factual. Separate factual conclusion from fanciful speculation.

Try not to use abbreviations in the concluding sentence; many readers look at the ***first*** and ***last*** sentences and then decide whether to read the entire abstract. Thus, it is important that these two sentences be completely clear. Be sure to leave your reader with a ***take-home message*** that ties in with your hypothesis.

Just the facts, Ma'am.

Lieutenant Joe Friday, *Dragnet* (1966)

Abstracts are important, but there are dangers in over-emphasizing them:

> *In an academic career, research and discovery are great fun; presenting the results of one's research in abstract form and having it accepted for presentation to a national society is even more fun; but writing the paper that the abstract is based on is often hell. Many people in academics have ruined their careers by devoting themselves to the 'fun' part and not the 'hell' part. My only advice is that the road to hell is paved with abstracts as far as an academic career is concerned.*
>
> William K. Schubert, M.D.
> Children's Hospital Medical Center
> Cincinnati, Ohio

Chapter 3

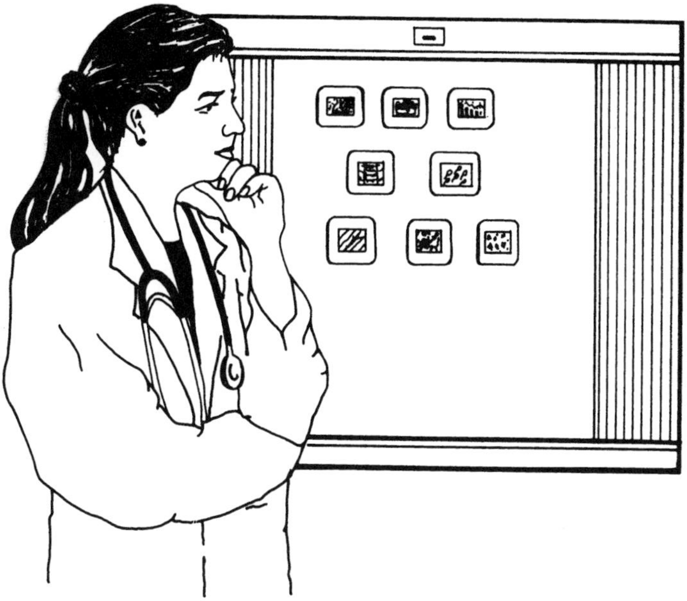

Making Effective Slides for a Lecture

3
Making Effective Slides for a Lecture

One picture is worth a thousand words.

Traditional Proverb

One man that has a mind and knows it, can always beat ten men who haven't and don't.

George Bernard Shaw
The Apple Cart (1929)

After your abstract has been accepted for presentation, one of the most exciting events in academic life is to prepare a scientific talk illustrated with slides. There are many pitfalls in this activity, and sitting through any scientific session at any meeting provides a good spectrum of the pitfalls that await the unwary.

Audience

Anticipate the needs of your audience by determining their knowledge of the topic, their interests and biases. Too few slides may make some of your audience restless as they lose their train of thought; zipping through too many slides will not give the audience enough time to digest each thought.

Preparation of Slides

Keep the slides simple. Condense the verbiage. Eliminate unnecessary details from graphs and charts. Be sure the slide is legible and visible from the ***back of a large room***. People who are sitting in the back are often less interested than those in the front; it is good not to lose them entirely! A rule of thumb is that a finished slide can be read by the naked eye at arm's length.

Label each slide with a ***simple title.*** Avoid abbreviations, if possible.

Lettering should be in ***capitals*** or bold type. Ordinary type results in letters that are too thin and cannot be seen from the back of the room.

If you are using tables (or text), ***do not use more than six lines;*** the maximum number of columns is also six. It is preferable to limit the rows or columns to four.

Label clearly the mean, ± SEM, r values, p values.

If you plan to use a standard computer to generate a graph, be careful. Standard computer print is often small and difficult to read on a slide. Use the arms-length test. In a big room the screen is usually not big enough for the people in the back to see.

Label the axes clearly on every graph and use the proper units. Axes should be ***interrupted*** if values do not go to zero or if there is a true interruption. Data points on graphs should not exceed the limits of numbers on the axes.

Regression lines on graphs should not be drawn to exceed the data points. Any ***extrapolation*** should be clearly identified, e.g., as dotted lines.

Avoid vertical slides. They are a problem because they inevitably project beyond the screen (unless you have a nimble projectionist with a zoom lens, a rare combination). One of the more embarrassing moments in presentations is the attempt to read slides projected on the ceiling or floor!

The Use of Color in Slides

White on black (black background with white lettering) is the sharpest and easiest to read in a large room with imperfectly dimmed lights. This combination is often so sharp that it can be read without dimming the lights. White on blue is the second (and prettier) choice. Because white on blue is less sharp, you must be even more careful about the use of small letters.

Use color to highlight the important features (graphs, tables, lettering), but do not overdo it. Use colors for contrast. On a dark background, ***use light colors;*** dark colors on a dark background (blue on black, for example) disappear. Against a dark background, yellow is best and orange is second best.

If you have access to a department of medical illustration, consider it a resource for producing slides of the highest quality. However, the scientific accuracy of the slides is your responsibility. Usually, you will provide drawings or sketches and graphs, which should be complete and accurate in every detail. The only responsibilities of the medical illustrator are to copy and beautify your artwork. After the medical illustrator has completed the drawings, make sure that you check them for accuracy very carefully before the slides are made.

Many excellent computer graphics programs permit you to make top-quality homemade slides. If you use such a program, remember that the listed guidelines are still important. The temptation to get carried away with all the options must be avoided. Do not include too much material or too many colors!

Presentation of a Talk with Slides

Use the following order:

- An introductory slide or two.
- A very specific hypothesis slide.
- A method slide.

- Results slides (the bulk of the presentation).
- Summary slides.
- A separate speculation slide listing one or two implications based on the data.

Ideally, have your slides in front of you while you are writing your speech. Make sure your text coincides with the slides so that the audience will be listening to you while reading the slides from left to right and from top to bottom. It is extremely distracting if your speech jumps from right to left or from bottom to top of a slide. Although some pages may be short, it saves a lot of trouble if your comments regarding each slide begin on a new page.

Practice the talk before ***as many critics as possible.*** Every rehearsal improves the presentation.

Start the talk with a few components that allow the audience to become familiar with your voice, accent, and cadence.

Introduce each slide. This gives the audience time to appreciate what is on the slide; they will then be ready to listen while you discuss the information on the slide.

Point out the axes of graphs for the audience; this also gives them more time to digest the data.

State and point to the ***specific relationship*** shown on the slide, e.g., "Y is significantly associated with X."

When presenting, ***provide enough time*** for the audience to view each slide. A good rule of thumb is to give 1½ minutes for each data slide and ½ minute for each nondata slide. The usual problem is that you will have too many slides. The novice always has two or three times as many slides as the veteran speaker.

When pointing with the electric pointer, do not keep the light on all the time. If you are trembling, the quivering light will be very obvious. If you are reading the text on the podium, it is easy to forget that your pointer light is still on, and its wanderings on the screen and ceiling will be distracting.

Point, do not circle with the light—unless you want to make your audience dizzy!

If the audience cannot read the slide, do not show it. Do not get into the habit of saying, "I know you can't read this slide, but . . . ."

Conclude each slide with a ***simple summary*** statement that indicates what one is supposed to learn from this slide.

Do not cram everything into your slides; the audience cannot absorb it. Save some for another talk.

Slides with complicated or very important information require double the usual viewing time. For such slides, go over each point carefully. For example, ratios are very difficult to follow; describe exactly what each numerator or denominator is.

At the end of your talk, leave the audience with a clear message: one or two major points, a maximum of three.

The Written Text That Supports Your Scientific Abstract Presentation

Because of limited time, the scientific abstract talk should be written out.

- Use simple sentences!
- Use LARGE CAPITALS and double space between lines in case the light over the lectern is dim or goes out.
- Keep the material for each slide on separate pages, so you will not need to turn a page while you are reading a slide.
- A suggestion: You may wish to keep your place in your manuscript with a finger on each line as you read, especially if you are using a pointer in the other hand.
- ***Bring your own pointer,*** if you can. Pointers at meetings fail 5% of the time, or may not even be available!
- Test the auditorium before the audience arrives.

- Run the slides once beforehand to see if they are in the right order, if the numbers match, if the correct side is up, if the projector is operating properly, and if the operator is competent. Practice your use of the pointer and slide controller before the audience arrives.

- Mark the lower left corner of each slide when you view it with the naked eye with a red dot; when you place the slides in the carousel, the red dot will then be on the upper right corner of all slides. This will help you or the operator to be sure they are loaded correctly.

- Number the slides so the operator will not fumble if they fall out. If available, lock the slides in place with the carousel lid.

How do I know what I think until I see what I say?

E. M. Forster (1922)

Question and Answer Period

At most scientific meetings, a question and answer period following each presentation is scheduled. Many young scientists, facing this exchange of information for the first time, experience acute anxiety because they do not know what the questions will be, and may be afraid of embarrassment for not knowing the answer. Even after some experience with this exchange, it is particularly disconcerting to see a senior member of a society with a reputation for intimidating younger scientists approach the microphone to ask a question. Do not panic but remember that there are many things in your favor; you have the data, he or she does not; you know the subject, he or she may not; you are a new investigator, he or she is an experienced person and the audience is generally on your side. Listen to the question carefully, answer clearly and directly, and if you do not know the answer, say so. The key to handling a question and answer session is to practice with your most supportive but toughest colleagues. Write down the key points of the questions; it helps keep you focused. A few choice extra slides can be very helpful. The more rehearsals the better.

Chapter 4

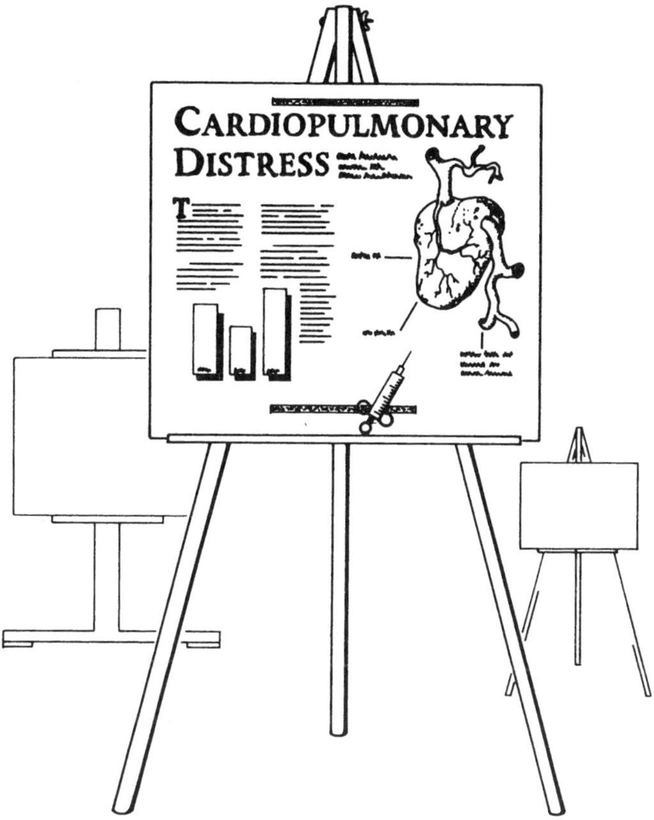

Giving Poster Presentations

4
Giving Poster Presentations

Ye see how large a letter I have written.

Galatians 6:11

Poster presentations are great opportunities for the young investigator. They provide an opportunity for you to stop (entrap?) a learned professor who is wandering by your poster and have him or her spend ten minutes, half an hour, or an hour with you, arguing about your methods, research design, or other specifics. This opportunity is rare at other occasions. This is also the best place to ***meet investigators*** in a similar field and to establish friendships that will last. Your ability to debate and think through solutions to your problems is enhanced through interactions such as these.

A few guidelines are helpful:

- The title should be large enough to be ***visible from fifteen feet.***
- The subtitles and important graphs should be visible from ten feet. With limited space, it is tempting to use smaller type for the title, subtitles, and graphs. This is an error because you are competing with others for the ***attention*** of an audience.

- ***Make everything graphic.*** This may be an impossible rule for some kinds of presentations, but using graphs instead of tables to present your whole message is the easiest way for your audience to see the ***relationship*** in your data.

- ***Avoid tables,*** if possible, especially tables that are filled with numbers, which are poorly received. If the use of such tables is unavoidable, make sure that key points are ***highlighted,*** so that the audience can find them easily.

- The logical order for the presentation of material is in columns from ***top to bottom*** and then in sequence from ***left to right.*** Use the panels like columns in a newspaper or journal. Do not have the text go all the way across the poster.

- A typical poster has ***seven sections:*** Abstract, Hypothesis, Introduction and Rationale, Methods, Results, Summary and Conclusion, and Speculation. Every poster need not have all seven, but if you omit one or add one, be sure you can justify doing so.

- ***Include the abstract of your work.*** If possible, have copies duplicated for distribution. Include in the handout the complete bibliographic description of the presentation and your name and professional address. A business card will come in handy.

- State the ***hypothesis*** clearly and simply.

- Present the ***introduction and rationale*** for your project for the broadest possible audience. As with all formal, scientific communication, a clear picture of your assumptions and intuitions about your project is essential in a poster presentation. The members of your audience who are most interested in your presentation will want to know the reasons you undertook this study and also why you chose your study design. You must provide this information for them.

- As you introduce the methods you used to demonstrate the validity of your hypothesis, if you used unique procedures or old procedures for new purposes, be sure to explain clearly exactly what you did.
- Itemize the results of your study clearly and concisely.
- Make sure the summary and conclusion of your presentation reflect the language and concepts of your hypothesis.
- Separate the unproved insights, the speculations, from the rest of the presentation. Most studies undertaken by an imaginative scientist will generate ideas and questions for further study and analysis. Such speculations are important and reflect the thoroughness of the study and the scientist's breadth of imagination.

> *Make it plain . . . so that he who runneth may read.*
>
> Habakkuk 2:2

Chapter 5

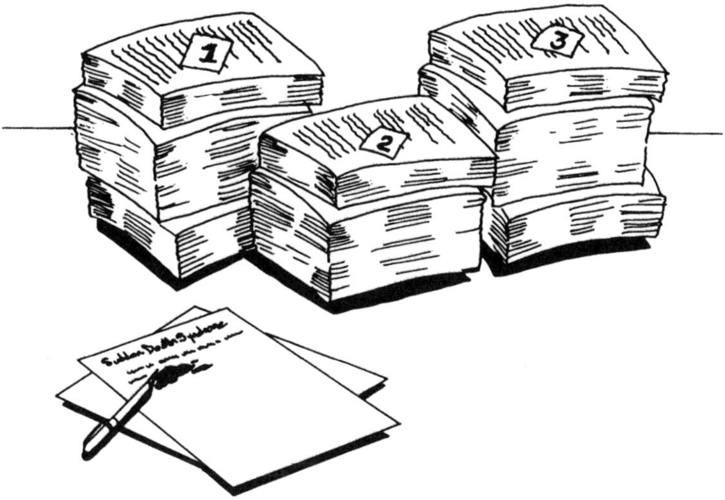

Writing an Original Paper

5
Writing an Original Paper

The only way to eat an elephant is one bite at a time.

Anonymous

When I am working on a book or a story, I write every morning as soon after the first light as possible. There is no one to disturb you and it is cool or cold and you come to your work and warm as you write.

Ernest Hemingway (1957)

To publish papers is one of the most important responsibilities of a scientist. Your publications demonstrate your career development and are also used to evaluate it. Publication is the gold standard against which most academic mettle is compared. By publishing, we sharpen our intellectual skills, we expose our data to critical review, and we may benefit society and the practice of medicine with our product. If your project is worth an abstract, it is probably ready to be developed into a manuscript. Your ideas are fresh in mind; they should be highly focused, and with additional effort and discipline, your abstract can become a manuscript. It is irresponsible to foist a half-baked abstract on an unsuspecting public if you are not prepared to defend your project by submitting your manuscript for peer review and publication.

Write the entire first draft in one sitting (ideally). If you try to write in spurts for several weeks or months, you might destroy your paper. The best approach is to "crash" a paper in one morning or afternoon. Do not let anyone or anything interfere with your thinking. Transform your thoughts into words as quickly and concisely as possible so you do not lose them. First make them concrete, then worry about polishing them.

> *Just get it down on paper, and then we'll see what to do with it.*
>
> Maxwell Perkins' advice
> to Marcia Davenport (1927)

Review the study proposal in which you listed all your hypotheses and keep a list of these major hypotheses before you as you write. This will help you to develop each section—introduction, methods, results, and discussion—in a ***logical*** sequence, corresponding to the hypotheses. We have all had the frustrating experience of trying to get to the point of a rambling paper. By keeping the ***main focus*** on your hypotheses, you may prevent this problem. This will allow your reader to follow the thought processes easily and logically. The reader wants to know what you set out to discover (specific hypotheses), how it was done (method), what was found (results), and how you came to your conclusions (discussion).

Organize. Bring together all the articles about which you think you want to write or comment. Decide to which hypothesis each article relates. ***Arrange the articles into separate stacks after you have read them once. Then begin to type or dictate at a fast pace.*** Beginning with the articles in stack one, summarize all points in reference to Hypothesis One; go to stack two to summarize points referring to Hypothesis Two, and so on. This system will help you to organize your reference materials logically.

Type or dictate at a fast rate to retain your train of thought. Do not worry about punctuation and grammar—those problems will be fixed when you edit subsequent drafts. After summarizing the points you wish to use from each article, dictate the names of the authors and the year of publication as a reminder. When you complete the paper, organize the references into their proper sequence.

You need not begin writing the paper with the introduction. Instead, put together all the data sections and begin wading immediately into your Results. These sections are among the easiest to write and should give you few problems. Then go back to write your Introduction. You can simply borrow some of the wording from your proposal. Next, move into your Discussion. As you have already covered the Methods section in your proposal, this section should be simple. Follow the sequence and the reasoning behind your ***original hypothesis*** exactly.

Send your paper to as many people as you can. Seeking honest input and constructive criticism is the best way to improve a paper. Someone looking at your paper from a different perspective can spot problems that you can easily rectify. ***Do not let your paper age on your desk for three months.*** Let comments serve as a ***provocation*** for you to keep the paper moving.

The concluding sentence is often the fatal one. Write it carefully. Your concluding sentence should be the one that addresses the key questions you raised in your hypotheses. You simply state the fact: "An increase in A resulted in a decrease in B." If you want to include a ***speculation,*** it should be phrased specifically as a speculation. Do not mix fact and fancy. When including speculation, state, "An increase in A resulted in a decrease in B; we speculate the reason for this is . . . ." Avoid the term "the data suggest," because semantically it is incorrect; ***you*** are suggesting, not the data—the data are the facts. Many articles have been lost because of the last line, and many misleading conclusions have been perpetrated on a gullible public.

Many of the concepts for writing review papers also can be applied to writing original papers, so take a look at Chapter 6, "Writing a Review Paper."

Authorship. Authors listed on the scientific paper should have been directly involved in the intellectual design of the study or the writing of the paper. Participants in the study who are fulfilling a technical role may be acknowledged in a footnote, but are not considered authors of the study. Primary authorship should be given to the person who has done the most work for the study and who has taken the initiative to write up the report and submit it for publication.

Chapter 6

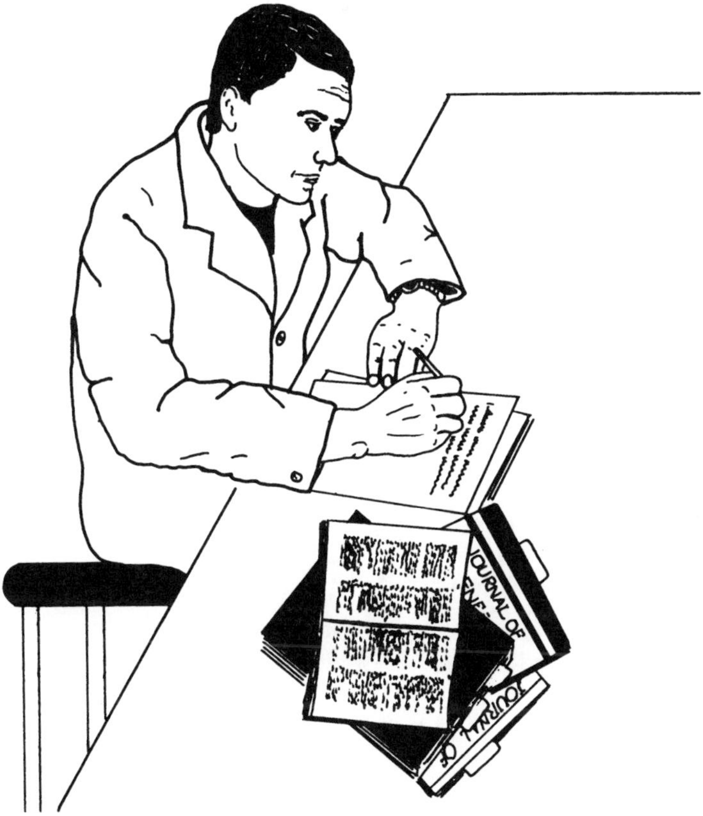

Writing a Review Paper

6
Writing a Review Paper

There's nothing to writing. All you do is sit down at a typewriter and open a vein.

Red Smith (1929)

Review papers give you the opportunity to be somewhat ***creative.*** When you write original articles, you will have many censors. But in a review paper, your conscience is often your only censor. As you synthesize these ideas and dreams, a pattern begins to emerge and a story begins to develop. Therefore, the ***story*** is the important issue.

Keep in mind that relative to your developing career, review papers should be a secondary priority. Review papers are not evidence of scientific productivity and have less bearing on academic promotion, grant applications, or membership in peer-reviewed societies. Review papers are often not peer-reviewed except in a few journals; therefore, their scientific value is less. They do, of course, have indirect scientific importance by educating many scientists who are usually outside your field of study.

If you do have the opportunity to write review papers early in your academic career, do so sparingly; make sure your time is well spent. Use the opportunity as a chance to focus on areas clearly relevant to your research. Furthermore, take advantage of the work you do to develop your next grant proposal (or vice versa).

Use the facts effectively to weave a coherent story.

Point out contradictions to your facts to provide balance, and allow the readers to draw some conclusions of their own. But do not get bogged down with contradictions. Your audience will lose track of your original story.

Be responsible for organizing all the facts logically. You are the expert who has been able to wade through a great deal of confusing information. After sifting through the morass of detail, you have a grasp of the entire story. Present your audience with the important issues.

Interpret the story and synthesize the studies for your audience. Do not list and summarize all the studies in the world. This process helps no one. A reader who wants to look closely at every study in the world will do so. Evaluate the studies critically and weave them together.

Be a ruthless critic. Not every study is important. Many are absolute rubbish. To quote them is to do the world a disservice, because such studies will continue to be perpetuated as if they are gospel! Root out the inept studies and use only those that you know are important.

Do NOT be too modest. Do not be ashamed to incorporate your own studies in your review paper. You know the data thoroughly. You know how precisely you have accumulated your data and specifically where the problems are. As the expert, you should be able to sift out the good from the bad in your own study. Your own studies enhance the quality of your paper by reflecting ***first-hand knowledge,*** as your studies confirm your authority. If you have no papers in the field, you should not be writing this review paper, unless you are writing one with a mentor who is established in the field.

Present your data in a logical sequence and be consistent in each section. For example:

- Each section might follow this pattern: animal data, adult data, childhood data, then infant data (that is, if you are writing a paper about infants).
- Move from relatively mundane to exciting descriptions to keep readers ***motivated*** and looking forward to reading on.
- Move from negative findings to positive findings. Punchlines should always be placed at the end; otherwise, readers will read right over them and not even realize they are there.

Use many diagrams and figures. A good picture is a feast for the eyes and can help the reader to understand your entire story. You will need to be creative with your drawings. Do not be discouraged if it takes several attempts to perfect your picture. Sketching out the visual parts of your article will also help you to focus on the important issues and sift out less important ones.

Include a summary statement at the conclusion of each section. Then, in the final conclusion, you can summarize the section summaries for an overall picture. The conclusion should not state any new facts, but should ***synthesize*** the summaries while leaving your reader with a message.

Chapter 7

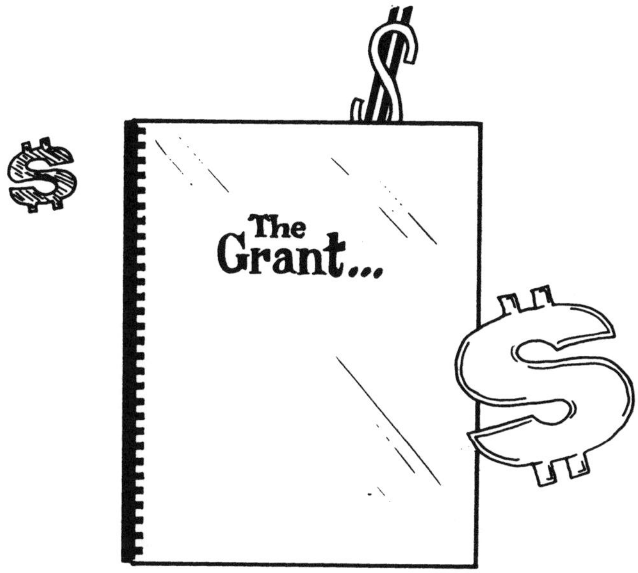

Writing a Grant Application

7
Writing a Grant Application

To write a grant application is one of the most important components of career development. The skills are among the highest intellectual skills in academic life, as they pit your wits against those of the best minds in your field. In essence, you are trying to convince a usually skeptical and usually sharp reviewer that your ideas are excellent and that investing in you will benefit science. To get funded not only provides autonomy for you, it also boosts your morale and enhances your credibility.

In the early years of your career, you may wish to avoid submitting grant applications to highly competitive organizations such as the National Institutes of Health or to national foundations with a highly rigorous peer review process. The reason for this caution is pragmatic: You will be competing with well-established, experienced investigators while your own scientific credibility is still unestablished. You might be better off during the first two or three post-fellowship years to concentrate your efforts on good, solid research funded by your own institution. This procedure may seem slow, but it will allow you to gain experience and to collect pilot data. You will also be able to publish a few of your manuscripts in peer-reviewed journals. These articles will help establish your credibility as a scientist when you begin writing major grant proposals.

In the meantime, you should submit grant applications to ***local affiliates*** of national foundations such as the American Heart Association, American Lung Association, March of Dimes, etc. These applications and the small grant awards will also give you the experience and confidence to apply for more highly competitive grants from national organizations later.

A grant application is like a ***debate.*** It is important to anticipate your opposition. Identify all the arguments your opponents may make, bring them out into the open, and demonstrate their weaknesses. Your opponents' arguments are weakened considerably because you have already identified and answered their challenges before they have opened their mouths. Your opposition in this debate is your reviewer, and you want to win. Any reviewer will try to "outsmart" you. If he or she outsmarts you, you are defeated this time, and you may have no chance to rebut.

Spend a great deal of time preparing your grant. Gather all the required supporting materials as soon as possible. Identify all possible problems and offer solutions. Review your application thoroughly, again and again.

State your goals clearly. As you write the purpose section of the grant, be sure your ***hypothesis*** is clear and concise. As you describe your goals, be specific and avoid broad categories that are vague and indecisive.

Have one, two, or three hypotheses. Do not try to list eighteen; you will never accomplish your goals. Alternatively, state a distinctive major hypothesis and one or two minor ones. Avoid the impression that you are going to conquer the world. Keep in mind that when you do twenty random analyses at one time, one of the analyses may be positive by chance. Therefore, be selective about the numbers of variables you intend to directly measure. By focusing on a few specific *a priori* hypotheses, you will be less liable to discover spuriously significant results.

Select the study design very carefully. Usually, the best clinical study design to convince cynics and critics is a ***longitudinal, randomized, double-blind study.*** Use this method as your reference point, and every time you depart from it, justify the deviation. It is your ***gold standard.*** In a longitudinal study, you are able to observe the chronological development of any subject. Such studies may take a long time, but your data will be useful and often unique.

Develop a focused argument. Write the opposing view first. If there is a defect in the opposition, point it out. The reviewer need not agree with you, but he or she does expect you to have thought through the problem. The reviewer is not looking for perfection but rather for a logical mind that has considered all aspects of the project. Be certain your thinking and your writing are ***logical and systematic.***

Anticipate a great deal of variation in clinical studies. Variations among individuals may overwhelm the differences you are seeking to find. Therefore, ***minimize as many variables as possible.*** Beginning with a clean population means that you will face dwindling numbers, but it is still the best way to undertake a clinical study. Investigators often mix apples and oranges to achieve larger numbers, but they lose a great deal of purity. Purity in this context means that your study is possibly going to be more difficult and take longer to complete, but the quality of your study will be enhanced. Thus, ***precise exclusions are important. Define your population well and discuss briefly the reasons for inclusion or exclusion of certain populations.***

Minimize the effects of biases. Bias kills many studies. Think ahead and plan your study carefully to reduce "flexibility" and opportunities for unknown biases. Frequently, technical staff are better at adhering to protocols; physicians are often tempted to be "flexible" and may subtly introduce biases.

Randomized study. The use of randomization in some studies is important to minimize the influence of unknown biases. If you undertake a randomized study, make sure that subject selection is truly random. Ideally, random assignment should be made by the use of random numbers. In practice, a coin toss might suffice. "Haphazard" selection, however, is not random selection and may introduce hidden biases.

Double-blind study. Most investigators have acquired unconscious biases over the years. Therefore, "blind" the observer, blind the subject, and blind the technicians. People may unconsciously believe they must prove a certain point; blinding helps eliminate this problem and ultimately can mean the success of your study. If for some reason you do not blind the study, be certain to indicate in your proposal why you do not propose to (or cannot) do so.

Use pair and other forms of matching. Matching is very important, and especially so in pediatrics. Gestational age, or age and gender, will often affect your results. Pair matching is tedious, and you will have smaller numbers, but the study may be much more accurate. Select from personal or previous studies what you know are the most powerful variables that affect what you are measuring. However, avoid matching for too many variables (such as more than three) to avoid proposing an impossible study. You cannot measure the factors you match; for example, you ***cannot*** determine whether race, gender, or age has an influence on the study if you match for these factors!

Assess all factors that will affect the measurements in your study. There are many factors that may affect your measurements. You need to determine those that are most important. Which ones make a difference? If you are writing a highly competitive grant proposal, it is good to include ***all*** factors, although you may not plan to study them nor be able to analyze the data, in which case just list them as other, unlikely possibilities. This will tell your reviewer that you have thought carefully about all aspects of your project.

Defend every test method you propose. Be precise. It is convenient and often very important to put the ongoing defense of the project in the Methods section. For example, each test method can be defended in that section according to how this particular measurement contributes to the testing of the hypotheses. ***Consider the frequency of measures.*** If you measure a subject many times, you will obviously have the opportunity to observe changes with time. However, repeated measures may invoke biases. Patients with the high values, for example, may become the most compliant subjects, returning regularly for examination; if this is the case, the higher frequency of sampling will bias the study. Be selective about the number of times patients are sampled. Ask yourself why you chose a special frequency. How does that frequency maximize the validity of your study?

Perform repeated measures-analyses on longitudinal studies. In longitudinal studies, measurements on each individual are repeatedly made. Because you have measured an event so many times, there is a one in twenty possibility that you will find a spuriously significant difference, using simple statistical analyses. Thus, statistical analyses that include adjustments for repeatedly measuring a variable within one subject should be applied.

Consider the times of sampling. Diurnal and other rhythms are often important. Be very strict about the times when you make your measures. Time of day, even the day of the week or month, may be significant factors to consider.

Use pilot studies to help convince grant reviewers. A pilot study shows you have the potential to complete the study and that you are aware of some of the pitfalls. In fact, NIH grants are rarely awarded without a pilot study.

> *Ideas are cheap; show me the data.*
>
> Reginald C. Tsang, M.D.
> University of Cincinnati
> Cincinnati, Ohio

Basic versus human studies. There is a myth among academicians that funding agencies with rigorous peer-review systems rarely support clinical research. Creative, well-designed, and well-written clinical proposals are funded, as long as the factors outlined earlier are carefully considered. Peer review groups in most funding agencies are quite aware of the difficulties surrounding clinical investigations and often take these difficulties into account in their review process.

Chapter 8

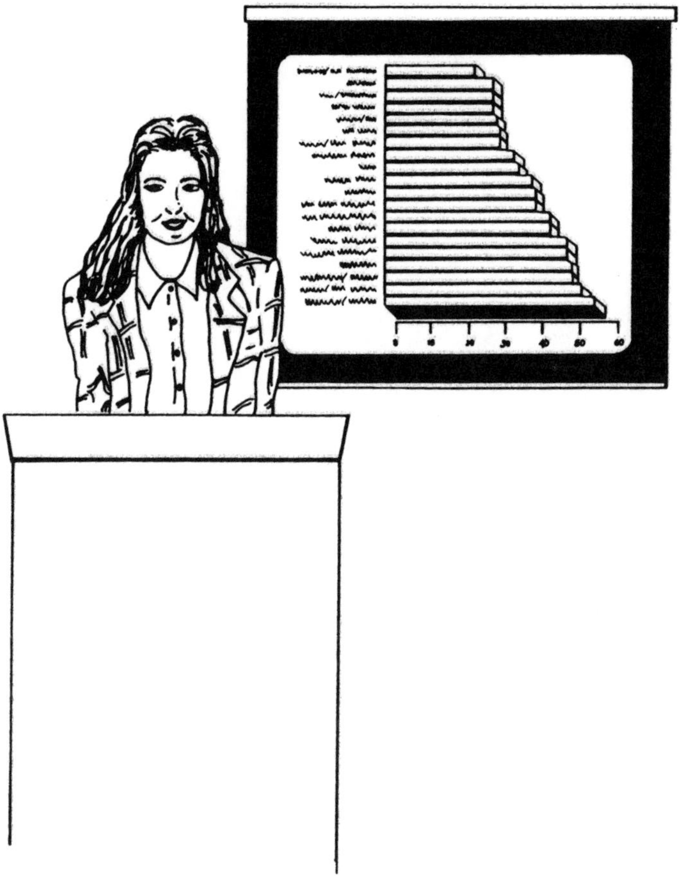

Presenting State-of-the-Art Lectures

8

Presenting State-of-the-Art Lectures

After you have established yourself as an authority with a good reputation, you will be invited to present a state-of-the-art or review-of-the-art lecture.

In the beginning of your career, try to accept invitations to speak regardless of the size and prestige of the meetings. Accepting invitations you receive (provided you perform well) frequently leads to other invitations. These invitations and speaking engagements allow you to improve your understanding of the subject, help your delivery, and (it is hoped) benefit others.

When the host asks for the title of your topic, make sure that the ***topic fits*** the interest of your audience. In clinical meetings, your topic should be relevant to the clinical practice of your audience. For instance, at a meeting of pediatricians in practice, topics such as antibiotics, treatment of sepsis, or management of birth asphyxia may be of greater interest than fluid and electrolyte management of very-low-birth-weight infants. In contrast, if you were to speak to neonatologists, the preference probably would be reversed.

If the sponsors of the meeting require a handout, prepare a good one, as this handout will be useful to augment your presentation. It could consist of a concise outline of some of the important slides that you show during your presentation. This will allow the audience to listen to you without the need to write down information.

Understand the composition of your audience. If you know what kind of people will be in your audience and what their interests are, your talk can be pitched precisely at them. If the audience is not made up of fellow experts, you must never be condescending. Ask the person who invited you who the audience is and what its previous experience with your topic is. Then prepare your talk accordingly.

Before your talk, get a sense of your audience by ***walking around*** and chatting with the people. In this way, you have an appreciation for exactly what they know and understand, and also what they expect. If possible, plan your itinerary so that you are at the meeting place ahead of schedule. You will have a chance to interact with some of your audience well before you speak, perhaps at a cocktail party the night before. This activity will always provide some interesting insights, especially if you are speaking in a foreign country.

Open with something interesting. Keep the talk interesting throughout the presentation by stressing unusual points, using visually interesting slides (see Chapter 3, "Making Effective Slides for a Lecture," page 19), and carefully adding personal anecdotes and jokes (if you are so inclined). Always allow enough time for the audience to review ***each*** slide (no faster than 1½ minutes per data slide).

Close with a bang if you can.

After you finish, anticipate a question and answer period, usually held at the end of each session. This period usually takes the form of a panel of the speakers. During this panel discussion, keep your responses as short as possible to allow time for other speakers. Be direct, helpful, and, if possible, diplomatic in your responses. Ask the audience occasionally to describe their experiences.

Chapter 9

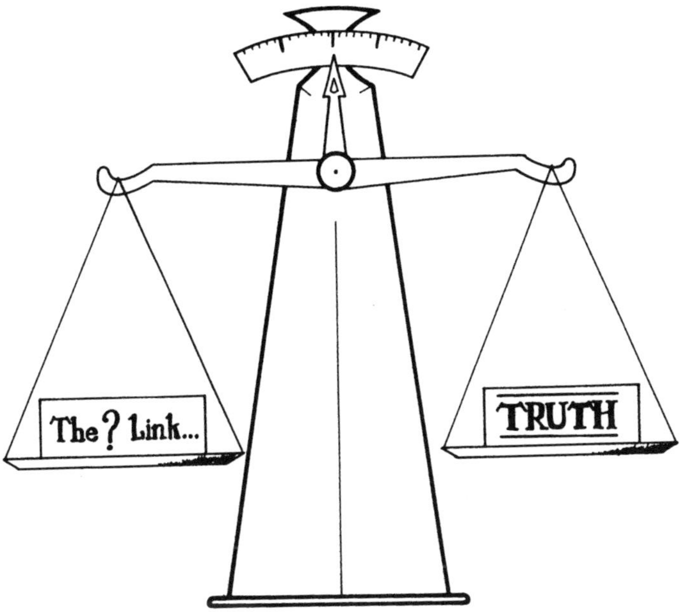

Understanding Fraud and Science

9
Understanding Fraud and Science

(Abstracted from Broad and Wade, *Betrayers of the Truth*, Simon and Schuster.)

Fraud in scientific research can occur at all stages of the process: when collecting data, when making an analysis, when interpreting analyses, and at the time of publication. The distinctions among error, bias, and fraud are narrow, and you can move almost innocently from error to bias and into fraud. Two basic causes of scientific fraud are self-deception and gullibility.

Self-Deception

Self-deception is a matter of seeing what we want to see. In Broad and Wade, two interesting cases are discussed: the famous mathematical horse, "Clever Hans," and his trainer and the case of the nonexistent "N-Rays."

Clever Hans was supposed to be able to count and perform simple arithmetic, tapping out the answers with his hoof. Hans impressed many learned people. But it turned out that the trainer was giving (presumably unconsciously) cues to the horse, so it would stop when it reached the correct number of hoof taps.

In 1902, the distinguished French physicist Rene Blondlot from the University of Nancy claimed to have discovered "N-Rays." Soon many other physicists reported seeing N-Rays. Blondlot discovered N-Rays in Broca's area in the brain when a person was talking, in magnetic fields, and in certain chemicals. The French Academy of Sciences awarded Blondlot the prestigious LeConte prize. A hundred scientists wrote, in 300 papers, that they had seen the effects of N-Rays. N-Rays were supposedly separated into different wavelengths after passing through a prism. An American physicist, R. W. Wood, visited Blondlot's laboratory and removed the prism before the experiment, but Blondlot claimed that he could still see the rays.

Gullibility

Magicians know that scientists are the easiest to fool because we want to believe. Our gullibility is our vulnerability and is best illustrated by the case of the Piltdown man. The Piltdown man was found to be a hoax a few decades after it was first "discovered." It consisted of an ape jaw with its molars filed down and a human skull stained to look aged.

Broad and Wade reported that a zoologist at the British Museum, suspicious about the Piltdown man, decided to perpetrate his own hoax. He took an ape tooth from the collection at the museum and filed it down; he took a leg bone from an extinct species of elephant, carved it into a "Pleistocene cricket bat," and buried all of the objects at Piltdown. Charles Dawson, the finder of the original Piltdown man, found these new diggings and was given additional credit, instead of ridicule!

Our conclusions from these stories are that because ***we see what we expect to see*** (we select the data that fit our hypothesis), and because we are the easiest to fool (we assume that all scientists are honest in describing their research), we should adopt the attitude that we should ***not trust the personal accuracy or honesty*** of any person describing his or her research. An individual may not be aware that he or she has slipped from error to bias or even to fraud. The individual could be self-deceived, and we could be gullible.

He must write as the interpreter of nature, and the legislator of mankind, and consider himself as presiding over the thoughts and manners of future generations; as being superior to time and place . . . . Integrity without knowledge is weak and useless, and knowledge without integrity is dangerous and dreadful.

Samuel Johnson (1759)

Chapter 10

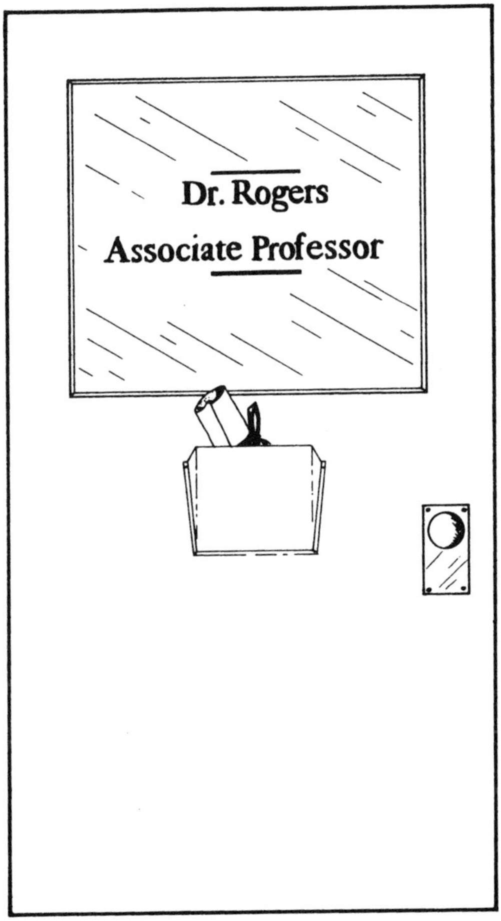

Getting an Academic Promotion

10
Getting an Academic Promotion

System of Appointment and Promotion

The young academician will begin a career as an instructor or assistant professor. At most universities, these initial appointments do not include tenure, but often lead to tenure and are called "tenure-track" appointments. Many colleges of medicine have a so-called 3-3-3 system, which means that an initial appointment is for three years, after which a candidate is reviewed for promotion, continuation, or termination. An assistant professor can be continued for up to two more three-year periods. At the end of the third three-year period, a candidate is either promoted to associate professor or advised to seek an alternate career. Appointments as associate professor in the academic track may include tenure.

> *A successful pediatric academician:*
>
> 1. *Remembers that he/she is a pediatrician who deals with a particular subspecialty in children and is not a subspecialist for children, and*
>
> 2. *Learns how to swim with the sharks.*
>
> John E. Lewy, M.D.
> Tulane Medical School
> New Orleans, Louisiana

Associate Professor

It may come as a surprise to many that one of the first requirements of the promotion process is that the candidate be a good and competent clinician. The next requirement is to be a good teacher. During clinical faculty rotations, students, house staff, and fellows often complete written evaluations. These written evaluations are made available to the promotion committee and become the basis for judging whether you are a good teacher. The promotion committee also takes into account your contribution to the medical community, including membership in various administrative committees within the university and in local and regional medical societies. Thus, if you have time, it might help to make some contributions in this area. Keep your own file of any written comments in regard to your work.

> *Teaching is an extraordinarily rewarding experience. You live your life in the lives of your students.*
>
> Harold Harrison, M.D.
> Johns Hopkins
> Baltimore Maryland

An extremely important part in the academic promotion process is, of course, the evaluation of scholarly activity. The committee will judge scholarly activity on the basis of publications; grants received; prestigious local, regional, and national committee appointments; and national reputation among peers.

The assessment of publications is based not only on their number but also on their quality, and is determined in part by the reputation of journals in which papers are published. Thus, you should aim high when you submit your papers for publication in peer-reviewed journals. Remember that most promotion committees will not look favorably on publication in the form of abstracts and book chapters. If non–peer-reviewed publications outnumber peer-reviewed papers, it will count against you. Case reports generally have less academic merit, unless they are well studied and identify a truly novel finding.

Another consideration is whether the publications were based on the research you completed during or after your fellowship years. Probably half the papers published in peer-reviewed journals of good quality should be based on work you performed during your fellowship, and the other half of work while you were an assistant professor. It is important that the list of publications shows that abstracts were published one or two years before the same materials were published in peer-reviewed journals, which demonstrates the validity of the data and shows that you do not let the grass grow under your feet. One or two review or invited articles in your area of interest provide the perspective that your credentials are solid enough for you to be an expert, qualified to provide a timely review of the subject.

> *To be a successful academician takes a number of unique attributes. These include, but are not limited to the tenacity of a bulldog, the diplomacy of a career politician, and the skin of a pachyderm. Patience remains a virtue, time management is critical, and a good sense of humor is essential.*
>
> Avroy A. Fanaroff, M.D.
> Rainbow Babies & Childrens Hospital
> Cleveland, Ohio

To obtain grants is important for promotion in most universities. However, because of the increasingly rigorous requirements for federally funded grants, this criterion is becoming more difficult to fulfill. To be funded by the NIH or other rigorously peer-reviewed, national-funding organizations usually assures promotion to associate professor. Someone without federal funding, however, may be promoted on the basis of other merits.

Appointments to prestigious regional and national committees and membership in academic societies with a peer-review process provide objective criteria that validate your academic credentials. In addition, requests to review papers for specific journals or grant applications indicate recognition of your academic reputation by others.

The promotion committee will ask for a list of people to write letters of recommendation on your behalf. Be sure that these people have a national reputation themselves, know you well enough to write a good evaluation, and are known to be fair and credible. Keep in mind that if one or two write a somewhat negative letter, your promotion may be in jeopardy.

> *I base my evaluation of a successful academician on a simple criterion: the accomplishments and recognition achieved by his/her students. A good academician will have personally contributed to the advancement of knowledge, published numerous papers, and perhaps achieved some personal recognition; but a great academician will have produced students who have become creative and successful in their own fields as a result of the stimulus they received to think independently and creatively, to recognize problems, and to develop their own solutions for them.*
>
> Jack Metcoff, M.S., M.D., M.P.H.
> University of Oklahoma
> Oklahoma City, Oklahoma

Professor

Once you are promoted to associate professor, your next academic goal is full professorship. To accomplish this, you must maintain your scholarly productivity by publishing important manuscripts in peer-reviewed journals, assume a major teaching or clinical responsibility in your division, and be invited to become a member of a significant, peer-reviewed society, a speaker at national and international meetings, and a visiting professor in another medical school. All of these activities will reflect your national and international reputation.

> *Honor a physician with the honor due him, . . .*
> *for the Lord hath created him.*
>
> Ecclesiasticus (Aprocrypha) 38.1

Chapter 11

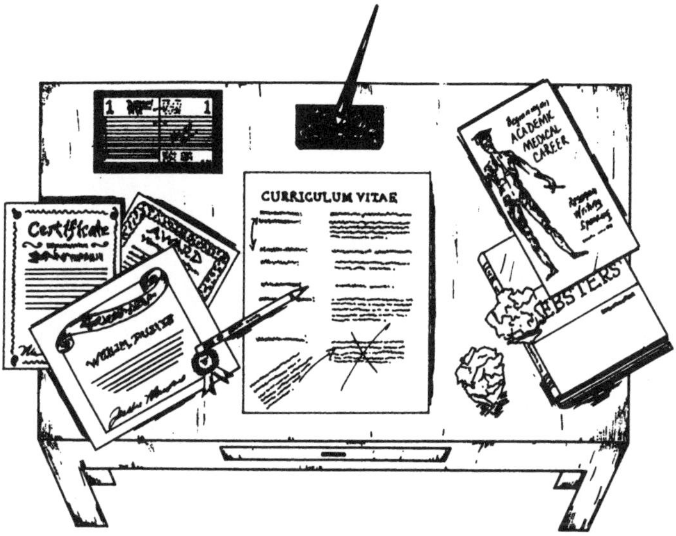

Preparing Your CV

11
Preparing Your Curriculum Vitae (CV)

In terms of education, training, and credentials, Sara Kelly, M.D., and Roy Cooper, M.D., were equally qualified for the position. Both had attended high-ranking medical schools and had served their residencies and fellowships under respected authorities in their field.

The position—at a major research hospital on the East coast—appealed to both young physicians as a major opportunity for professional advancement. Sara was among the final candidates interviewed at the hospital and eventually received the appointment. Roy was eliminated almost immediately—and did not understand why.

Sara's edge—and Roy's failure—came from the same source: the curriculum vitae (CV). Their story, with minor variations, will be repeated many times during the 90s, a decade of increased competition among young physicians at the beginning of their careers.

Because many hospitals and clinics—particularly those in the most desirable geographical locations—have more than enough qualified candidates for any position, the screening process begins immediately. And one of the first steps in applying for any position is preparation of the CV. Sara's CV was accurate, complete, and carefully prepared;

it demonstrated attention to detail, ability to organize, and professional commitment.

Roy, on the other hand, submitted a CV that he had thrown together in less than an hour, without checking for consistency, grammar, spelling, or style. In his haste he even omitted relevant details about awards and publications and gave incomplete information about his work experience.

But the physician director didn't even need to look closely at Roy's CV to know that it had been hastily prepared. Instead of composing his CV on a computer and generating a large supply of originals, Roy relied on a photocopier at the hospital. The result was blurred and hard to read.

Too often, young physicians follow the example of Roy rather than Sara. They forget that, no matter how qualified they may be, the first step is to get their foot in the door. Marketing has become a major aspect of the medical profession, and candidates for any position must carefully market themselves—to the physician director, to the hospital administrator, even to a governing board.

The CV requires a great deal of ***advance planning*** that, ideally, should begin the year before completion of the fellowship. This time frame allows the opportunity to review and modify the resume, so that the final form is professional and polished.

The first rule, of course, is to be honest. Embellishments have a way of backfiring and discrediting even the truth. The people who review CVs have readily available resources to check reported information.

The second rule is to ensure that the information is complete. Obviously the CV should summarize education, training, and work experience; but it should also highlight other accomplishments, such as awards, honors, and publications, and provide a brief overview of special skills and interests.

The format should be consistent throughout. Summaries may be organized in chronological or reverse chronological order or even by abilities and skills. A combination of strategies is often advisable, but overall organization should never seem random or arbitrary. Consistency of format from section to section makes the CV easy to follow and easy to compare.

Whatever format is adopted, every CV should include the following vital information:

Full name, home address, and home telephone number.

Work telephone and fax number. Listing the best time and place to call is often a good idea if your schedule is particularly hectic.

Education. Generally undergraduate work is listed first, followed by postgraduate training, medical school, internship, residency, and fellowship. Be sure to include dates, locations, and degrees received at each institution.

Certification and licensure. Specialty status—board certified or board eligible—should be clearly indicated, along with pertinent dates and jurisdictions. It is standard to include dates and types of licensure exams, but unnecessary to include scores.

Professional experiences. Research projects, teaching and administrative assignments, and even extra medical jobs should be included, particularly if they fill in the gaps in education or training. It is standard procedure to list them in chronological order, giving relevant addresses, dates, and descriptions of duties.

Awards, honors, professional memberships. Appropriate awards and honors should be listed in chronological order. Professional societies should be listed in the order in which they were joined, along with specific dates of membership.

Publications/presentations. Standard bibliographical form and chronological order should be used.

Personal information. Special skills and hobbies, including nonmedical activities and interests, should be selectively listed. For example, fluency in a foreign language and volunteer work for a charitable or civic group may be appropriate; a passion for hang-gliding usually is not! Choose carefully.

References. Listing the names of specific references is optional. Some experts advise against it and recommend instead use of the standard phrase, "Available upon request." This strategy allows choice of the most appropriate references for each situation and prevents wasting the time of mentors, bosses, and colleagues on phone calls or letters for positions that are third or fourth rather than first or second choices. Other experts argue that listing the names of well-known experts as references makes a CV stand out by drawing immediate attention to the quality of the candidate. Practicality suggests that this strategy is appropriate for highly desired or highly competitive positions. Whichever strategy is used, the list should include two or three professional references, often including the director of the candidate's fellowship or residency program.

Preparation of the CV also involves a certain number of taboos. Salary requirements should never be listed unless specifically requested, and photographs usually should not be included. The first is unconventional and creates an unnecessary barrier by implying that the candidate is inflexible; unless requested, the second may lead to judgment based on appearance rather than qualifications.

Common sense dictates that the CV should be clean as well as legible, without lipstick or coffee stains on the copy! A properly addressed letter should accompany the CV. "To whom it may concern" is not an acceptable salutation; use the name(s) of the person(s) to whom the CV is submitted. The letter itself should be short and to the point, specifying the position for which the candidate is applying and, if appropriate, how the position came to the candidate's attention. A brief description of the candidate's current affiliation is standard, but details of education, training, and work experience should be reserved for the CV.

As a final tip, it is often beneficial for the inexperienced candidate to search out a copy of the CV of a distinguished senior professor or authority in the same field. Professional models are often a major source of inspiration—but don't be too surprised if the CV of a Nobel prize winner breaks all the rules and violates all the taboos. In that case, look for another model that is more appropriate for the first-time candidate.

Careful preparation of the CV is more than an exercise in format and protocol. The CV is an important document that should be regularly updated throughout a physician's career. In addition to employment purposes, it is also necessary for joining medical organizations; applying for licensure; and obtaining hospital privileges, among many other tasks. The well-prepared CV sets the stage for an academic medical career.

Appendix

Uniform Requirements for Manuscripts Submitted to Biomedical Journals

International Committee of Medical Journal Editors

Fourth Edition

In January 1978 a group of editors from some major biomedical journals published in English met in Vancouver, British Columbia, and decided on uniform technical requirements for manuscripts to be submitted to their journals. These requirements, including formats for bibliographic references developed for the Vancouver group by the National Library of Medicine, were published in three of the journals early in 1979. The Vancouver group evolved into the International Committee of Medical Journal Editors. Over the years, the group has revised the requirements slightly; this is the fourth edition.

Over 400 journals have agreed to receive manuscripts prepared in accordance with the requirements. It is important to emphasize what these requirements imply and what they do not.

First, the requirements are instructions to authors on how to prepare manuscripts, not to editors on publication style. (But many journals have drawn on these requirements for elements of their publication styles.)

Second, if authors prepare their manuscripts in the style specified in these requirements, editors of the participating journals will not return manuscripts for changes in these details of style. Even so, manuscripts may be altered by journals to conform with details of their own publication styles.

Third, authors sending manuscripts to a participating journal should not try to prepare them in accordance with the publication style of that journal but should follow the "Uniform Requirements for Manuscripts Submitted to Biomedical Journals."

Nevertheless, authors must also follow the instructions to authors in the journal as to what topics are suitable for that journal and the types of papers that may be submitted—for example, original articles, reviews, or case reports. In addition, the journal's instructions are likely to contain other requirements unique to that journal, such as number of copies of manuscripts, acceptable languages, length of articles, and approved abbreviations.

Participating journals are expected to state in their instructions to authors that their requirements are in accordance with the "Uniform Requirements for Manuscripts Submitted to Biomedical Journals" and to cite a published version.

This document will be revised at intervals. Inquiries and comments from Central and North America about these requirements should be sent to Editor, the *New England Journal of Medicine,* 10 Shattuck St., Boston, MA 02115; those from other regions should be sent to Editor, *British Medical Journal,* British Medical Association, Tavistock Sq., London WC1H 9JR, United Kingdom. Note that these two journals provide secretariat services for the International Committee of Medical Journal Editors; they do not handle manuscripts intended for other journals. Papers intended for other journals should be sent directly to the offices of those journals.

Summary of Requirements

Type the manuscript double-spaced, including title page, abstract, text, acknowledgments, references, tables, and legends.

Each manuscript component should begin on a new page, in the following sequence: title page; abstract and key words; text; acknowledgments; references; tables (each table complete with title and footnotes on a separate page); and legends for illustrations.

Illustrations must be good-quality, unmounted glossy prints, usually 127 × 173 mm (5 × 7 in.), but no larger than 203 × 254 mm (8 × 10 in.).

Submit the required number of copies of manuscript and figures (see journal's instructions) in a heavy paper envelope. The submitted manuscript should be accompanied by a covering letter, as described under Submission of Manuscripts, and permissions to reproduce previously published material or to use illustrations that may identify human subjects.

Follow the journal's instructions for transfer of copyright. Authors should keep copies of everything submitted.

Prior and Duplicate Publication

Most journals do not wish to consider for publication a paper on work that has already been reported in a published paper or is described in a paper submitted or accepted for publication elsewhere. This policy does not usually preclude consideration of a paper that has been rejected by another journal or of a complete report that follows publication of a preliminary report, usually in the form of an abstract. Nor does it prevent consideration of a paper that has been presented at a scientific meeting if not published in full in a proceedings or similar publication. Press reports of the meeting will not usually be considered as breaches of this rule, but such reports should not be amplified by additional data or copies of tables and illustrations. When submitting a paper an author should always make a full statement to the editor about all submissions and previous reports that might be regarded as prior or duplicate publication of the same or very similar work. Copies of such material should be included with the submitted paper to help the editor decide how to deal with the matter.

Multiple publication—that is, the publication more than once of the same study, irrespective of whether the wording is the same—is rarely justified. Secondary publication in another language is one possible justification, provided the following conditions are met.

(1) The editors of both journals concerned are fully informed; the editor concerned with secondary publication should have a photocopy, reprint, or manuscript of the primary version.

(2) The priority of the primary publication is respected by a publication interval of at least two weeks.

(3) The paper for secondary publication is written for a different group of readers and is not simply a translated version of the primary paper; an abbreviated version will often be sufficient.

(4) The secondary version reflects faithfully the data and interpretations of the primary version.

(5) A footnote on the title page of the secondary version informs readers, peers, and documenting agencies that the paper was edited, and is being published, for a national audience in parallel with a primary version based on the same data and interpretations. A suitable footnote might read as follows: "This article is based on a study first reported in the [title of journal, with full reference]."

Multiple publication other than as defined above is not acceptable to editors. If authors violate this rule they may expect appropriate editorial action to be taken.

Preliminary release, usually to public media, of scientific information described in a paper that has been accepted but not yet published is a violation of the policies of many journals. In a few cases, and only by arrangement with the editor, preliminary release of data may be acceptable—for example, to warn the public of health hazards.

Preparation of Manuscript

Type the manuscript on white bond paper, 216 × 279 mm (8 × 11 in.) or ISO A4 (212 × 297 mm), with margins of at least 22 mm (1 in.). Type only on one side of the paper. Use double-spacing throughout, including title page, abstract, text, acknowledgments, references, tables, and legends for illustrations. Begin each of the following sections on separate pages: title page, abstract and key words, text, acknowledgments, references, individual tables, and legends. Number pages consecutively, beginning with the title page. Type the page number in the upper or lower right-hand corner of each page.

Title Page

The title page should carry (a) the title of the article, which should be concise but informative; (b) first name, middle initial, and last name of each author, with highest academic degree(s) and institutional affiliation; (c) name of department(s) and institution(s) to which the work should be attributed; (d) disclaimers, if any; (e) name and address of author responsible for correspondence about the manuscript; (f) name and address of author to whom requests for reprints should be addressed or statement that reprints will not be available from the author; (g) source(s) of support in the form of grants, equipment, drugs, or all of these; and (h) a short running head or foot line of no more than 40 characters (count letters and spaces) placed at the foot of the title page and identified.

Authorship

All persons designated as authors should qualify for authorship. The order of authorship should be a joint decision of the coauthors. Each author should have participated sufficiently in the work to take public responsibility for the content.

Authorship credit should be based only on substantial contributions to (a) conception and design, or analysis and interpretation of data; and to (b) drafting the article or revising it critically for important intellectual content; and on (c) final approval of the version to be published. Conditions (a), (b), and (c) must all be met. Participation solely in the acquisition of funding or the collection of data does not justify authorship. General supervision of the research group is also not sufficient for authorship. Any part of an article critical to its main conclusions must be the responsibility of at least one author.

A paper with corporate (collective) authorship must specify the key persons responsible for the article; others contributing to the work should be recognized separately (see Acknowledgments).

Editors may require authors to justify the assignment of authorship.

Abstract and Key Words

The second page should carry an abstract (of no more than 150 words for unstructured abstracts or 250 words for structured abstracts). The abstract should state the purposes of the study or investigation, basic procedures (selection of study subjects or laboratory animals; observational and analytical methods), main findings (give specific data and their statistical significance, if possible), and the principal conclusions. Emphasize new and important aspects of the study or observations.

Below the abstract provide, and identify as such, 3 to 10 key words or short phrases that will assist indexers in cross-indexing the article and may be published with the abstract. Use terms from the medical subject headings (MeSH) list of *Index Medicus;* if suitable MeSH terms are not yet available for recently introduced terms, present terms may be used.

Text

The text of observational and experimental articles is usually—but not necessarily—divided into sections with the headings Introduction, Methods, Results, and Discussion. Long articles may need subheadings within some sections to clarify their content, especially the Results and Discussion sections. Other types of articles such as case reports, reviews, and editorials are likely to need other formats. Authors should consult individual journals for further guidance.

Introduction. State the purpose of the article. Summarize the rationale for the study or observation. Give only strictly pertinent references, and do not review the subject extensively. Do not include data or conclusions from the work being reported.

Methods. Describe your selection of the observational or experimental subjects (patients or laboratory animals, including controls) clearly. Identify the methods, apparatus (manufacturer's name and address in parentheses), and procedures in sufficient detail to allow other workers to reproduce the results. Give references to established methods, including statistical methods (see below); provide references and brief descriptions for methods that have been published but are not well known; describe new or substantially modified methods, give reasons for using them, and evaluate their limitations. Identify precisely all drugs and chemicals used, including generic name(s), dose(s) and route(s) of administration.

Ethics. When reporting experiments on human subjects indicate whether the procedures followed were in accordance with the ethical standards of the responsible committee on human experimentation (institutional or regional) or with the Helsinki Declaration of 1975, as revised in 1983. Do not use patients' names, initials, or hospital numbers, especially in any illustrative material. When reporting experiments on animals indicate whether the institution's or the National Research Council's guide for, or any national law on, the care and use of laboratory animals was followed.

Statistics. Describe statistical methods with enough detail to enable a knowledgeable reader with access to the original data to verify the reported results. When possible, quantify findings and present them with appropriate indicators of measurement error or uncertainty (such as confidence intervals). Avoid sole reliance on statistical hypothesis testing, such as the use of P values, which fails to convey important quantitative information. Discuss eligibility of experimental subjects. Give details about randomization. Describe the methods for and success of any blinding observations. Report treatment complications. Give numbers of observations. Report losses to observation (such as dropouts from a clinical trial). References for study design and statistical methods should be to standard works (with pages stated) when possible rather than to papers in which the designs or methods were originally reported. Specify any general-use computer programs used.

Put general descriptions of methods in the Methods section. When data are summarized in the Results section specify the statistical methods used to analyze them. Restrict tables and figures to those needed to explain the argument of the paper and to assess its support. Use graphs as an alternative to tables with many entries; do not duplicate data in graphs and tables. Avoid nontechnical uses of technical terms in statistics, such as "random" (which implies a randomizing device), "normal," "significant," "correlations," and "sample." Define statistical terms, abbreviations, and most symbols.

Results. Present your results in logical sequence in the text, tables, and illustrations. Do not repeat in the text all the data in the tables or illustrations; emphasize or summarize only important observations.

Discussion. Emphasize the new and important aspects of the study and the conclusions that follow from them. Do not repeat in detail data or other material given in the Introduction or the Results section. Include in the Discussion section the implications of the findings and their limitations, including implications for future research. Relate the observations to other relevant studies. Link the conclusions with the goals of the study but avoid unqualified statements and conclusions not completely supported by your data. Avoid claiming priority and alluding to work that has not been completed. State new hypotheses when warranted, but clearly label them as such. Recommendations, when appropriate, may be included.

Acknowledgments

At an appropriate place in the article (title-page footnote or appendix to the text; see the journal's requirement) one or more statements should specify (a) contributions that need acknowledging but do not justify authorship, such as general support by a departmental chairman; (b) acknowledgments of technical help; (c) acknowledgments of financial and material support, specifying the nature of the support; (d) financial relationships that may pose a conflict of interest.

Persons who have contributed intellectually to the paper but whose contributions do not justify authorship may be named and their function or contribution described—for example, "scientific adviser," "critical review of study proposal," "data collection," or "participation in clinical trial." Such persons must have given their permission to be named. Authors are responsible for obtaining written permission from persons acknowledged by name, because readers may infer their endorsement of the data and conclusions.

Technical help should be acknowledged in a paragraph separate from those acknowledging other contributions.

References

Number references consecutively in the order in which they are first mentioned in the text. Identify references in text, tables, and legends by Arabic numerals in parentheses. References cited only in tables or in legends to figures should be numbered in accordance with a sequence established by the first identification in the text of the particular table or illustration.

The titles of journals should be abbreviated according to the style used in *Index Medicus*. Consult *List of Journals Indexed in Index Medicus*, published annually as a separate publication by the National Library of Medicine (8 600 Rockville Pike, Bethesda, MD 20894), and as a list in the January issue of *Index Medicus*.

Try to avoid using abstracts as references; "unpublished observations" and "personal communications" may not be used as references, although references to written, not oral, communications may be inserted (in parentheses) in the text. Include among the references papers accepted but not yet published; designate the journal and add "In press." Information from manuscripts submitted but not yet accepted should be cited in the text as "unpublished observations" (in parentheses).

The references must be verified by the author(s) against the original documents.

Tables

Type each table double-spaced on a separate sheet. Do not submit tables as photographs. Number tables consecutively in the order of their first citation in the text and supply a brief title for each. Give each column a short or abbreviated heading. Place explanatory matter in footnotes, not in the heading. Explain in footnotes all nonstandard abbreviations that are used in each table. For footnotes use the following symbols, in this sequence: *, †, ‡, §, ||, ¶, **, ††, ...

Identify statistical measures of variations such as standard deviation and standard error of the mean.

Do not use internal horizontal and vertical rules.

Be sure that each table is cited in the text.

If you use data from another published or unpublished source, obtain permission and acknowledge fully.

The use of too many tables in relation to the length of the text may produce difficulties in the layout of pages. Examine issues of the journal to which you plan to submit your paper to estimate how many tables can be used per 1000 words of text.

The editor, on accepting a paper, may recommend that additional tables containing important backup data too extensive to publish be deposited with an archival service, such as the National Auxiliary Publication Service in the United States, or made available by the authors. In that even an appropriate statement will be added to the text. Submit such tables for consideration with the paper.

Illustrations

Submit the required number of complete sets of figures. Figures should be professionally drawn and photographed; freehand or typewritten lettering is unacceptable. Instead of original drawings, roentgenograms, and other material, send sharp, glossy black-and-white photographic prints, usually 127 × 173 mm (5 × 7 in.), but no larger than 203 × 254 mm (8 × 10 in.). Letters, numbers, and symbols should be clear and even throughout and of sufficient size that when reduced for publication each item will still be legible. Titles and detailed explanations belong in the legends for illustrations, not on the illustrations themselves.

Each figure should have a label pasted on its back indicating the number of the figure, author's name, and top of the figure. Do not write on the back of figures or scratch or mar them by using paper clips. Do not bend figures or mount them on cardboard.

Photomicrographs must have internal scale markers. Symbols, arrows, or letters used in the photomicrographs should contrast with the background.

If photographs of persons are used, either the subjects must not be identifiable or their pictures must be accompanied by written permission to use the photograph.

Figures should be numbered consecutively according to the order in which they have been first cited in the text. If a figure has been published, acknowledge the original source and submit written permission from the copyright holder to reproduce the material. Permission is required irrespective of authorship or publisher, except for documents in the public domain.

For illustrations in color, ascertain whether the journal requires color negatives, positive transparencies, or color prints. Accompanying drawings marked to indicate the region to be reproduced may be useful to the editor. Some journals publish illustrations in color only if the author pays for the extra cost.

Legends for Illustrations

Type legends for illustrations double-spaced, starting on a separate page, with Arabic numerals corresponding to the illustrations. When symbols, arrows, numbers, or letters are used to identify parts of the illustrations, identify and explain each one clearly in the legend. Explain the internal scale and identify method of staining in photomicrographs.

Units of Measurement

Measurements of length, height, weight, and volume should be reported in metric units (meter, kilogram, or liter) or their decimal multiples.

Temperatures should be given in degrees Celsius. Blood pressures should be given in millimeters of mercury.

All hematologic and clinical-chemistry measurements should be reported in the metric system in terms of the International System of Units (SI). Editors may request that alternative or non-SI units be added by the authors before publication.

Abbreviations and Symbols

Use only standard abbreviations. Avoid abbreviations in the title and abstract. The full term for which an abbreviation stands should precede its first use in the text unless it is a standard unit of measurement.

Submission of Manuscripts

Mail the required number of manuscript copies in a heavy paper envelope, enclosing the manuscript copies and figures in cardboard, if necessary, to prevent bending of photographs during mail handling. Place photographs and transparencies in a separate heavy paper envelope.

Manuscripts must be accompanied by a covering letter signed by all coauthors. This must include (a) information on prior or duplicate publication or submission elsewhere of any part of the work as defined earlier in this document;

(b) a statement of financial or other relationships that might lead to a conflict of interest; (c) a statement that the manuscript has been read and approved by all authors, that the requirements for authorship as previously stated in this document have been met, and furthermore, that each coauthor believes that the manuscript represents honest work; and (d) the name, address, and telephone number of the corresponding author, who is responsible for communicating with the other authors about revisions and final approval of the proofs. The letter should give any additional information that may be helpful to the editor, such as the type of article in the particular journal the manuscript represents and whether the author(s) will be willing to meet the cost of reproducing color illustrations.

The manuscript must be accompanied by copies of any permissions to reproduce published material, to use illustrations or report sensitive personal information of identifiable persons, or to name persons for their contributions.

Participating Journals

Journals that have notified the International Committee of Medical Journal Editors of their willingness to consider for publication manuscripts prepared in accordance with earlier versions of the committee's uniform requirements identify themselves as such in their information for authors. A full list is available on request from the *New England Journal of Medicine* or the *British Medical Journal*. Citations of this document should be to one of the sources listed below.

International Committee of Medical Journal Editors. Uniform requirements for manuscripts submitted to biomedical journals. N Engl J Med 1991; 324:424–8.

International Committee of Medical Journal Editors. Uniform requirements for manuscripts submitted to biomedical journals. BMJ 1991; 302;338–41.

Widely cited guidelines for medical scientific publications by the International Committee for Medical Journal Editors are found on the web at www.icmje.org.

Recommended Reading

Abels FB: *How to Prepare an Effective Scientific Research Proposal.* Philadelphia, ISI Press, 1985.

American Medical Association: *Manual of Style,* 8th ed. Baltimore, Williams & Wilkins, 1989.

American Society for Microbiology: *ASM Style Manual for Journals and Books.* Washington, DC, American Society for Microbiology, 1985.

Armitage P: *Statistical Methods in Medical Research.* New York, NY, Halsted Press, 1971.

Barrars R: *Scientists Must Write: A Quick Guide to Better Writing for Scientists.* New York, Wiley, 1978.

Bernstein TM: *The Careful Writer: A Modern Guide to English Usage.* New York, NY, Atheneum, 1984.

Booth VH: *Writing a Scientific Paper and Speaking at Scientific Meetings,* 5th ed. London, Biochemical Society, 1981.

Brownlee KA: *Statistical Theory and Methodology in Science and Engineering,* 2nd ed. New York, NY, John Wiley & Sons Inc., 1965.

CBE Style Manual Committee: *CBE Style Manual: A Guide for Authors, Editors, and Publishers in the Biological Sciences,* 5th ed. Bethesda, MD, Council of Biology Editors Inc., 1983.

The Chicago Manual of Style, 13th ed. Chicago, IL, University of Chicago Press, 1982.

Clements W: *The Scientific Report: A Guide for Authors.* San Diego, Society for Technical Communications, 1984.

Cochran WG: *Sampling Techniques,* 2nd ed. New York, NY, John Wiley & Sons Inc., 1963.

Cochran WG, Cox GM: *Experimental Designs,* 2nd ed. New York, NY, John Wiley & Sons Inc., 1957.

Colton T: *Statistics in Medicine.* Boston, MA, Little Brown & Co., Inc., 1974.

Day RA: *How to Write and Publish a Scientific Paper,* 3rd ed. Phoenix, AZ, Oryx Press, 1988.

Dodd JS (ed): *The ACS Style Guide: A Manual for Authors and Editors.* Washington, DC, American Chemical Society, 1985.

Feinstein AR: *Clinical Epidemiology: The Architecture of Clinical Research.* Philadelphia, PA, W.B. Saunders Co., 1985.

Fishbein M: *Medical Writing: The Technic and the Art,* 4th ed. Springfield, IL, Charles C Thomas Publisher, 1978.

Fleiss J: *Statistical Methods for Rates and Proportions,* 2nd ed. New York, NY, John Wiley & Sons Inc., 1981.

Halls M: *Developing Skills in Proposal Writing,* 2nd ed. Portland, OR, Continuing Education Publications, 1977.

Hawkins C, Sorgi M (eds): *Research: How to Plan, Speak and Write About It.* Berlin, West Germany, Springer-Verlag, 1985.

Hulley and Cummings: *Designing Clinical Research.* Baltimore, Williams & Wilkins, 1988.

Huth EJ: *How to Write and Publish Papers in the Medical Sciences,* 2nd ed. Baltimore, Williams & Wilkins, 1990.

Huth EJ: *Medical Style & Format: An International Manual for Authors, Editors, and Publishers.* Philadelphia, PA, ISI Press, 1987.

Jablonski S: *Dictionary of Medical Acronyms and Abbreviations,* 2nd ed. Philadelphia, Hanley & Belfus, 1993.

King LS: *Why Not Say It Clearly: A Guide to Scientific Writing.* Boston, MA, Little Brown & Co. Inc., 1978.

Kiritz NJ: *Proposal Checklist and Evaluation Forms.* Los Angeles, CA, Grantsmanship Center, 1979.

McMaster University: "Academic Medicine." *Canadian Medical Association Journal* 124:555–558, 703–710, 869–872, 1156–1161, 1981.

Orlich DC: *The Art of Writing Successful Research and Development Proposals.* Pleasantville, NY, Redgrave Publishing, 1977.

Roland CG: *Good Scientific Writing: An Anthology.* Chicago, AMA Press, 1971.

Snedecor GW, Cochran WG: *Statistical Methods,*7th ed. Ames, IA, Iowa State University Press, 1980.

Steen MD: *Instructions for Authors: Biomedical Journals.* Orlando, Academic Press, 1985.

Strunk W Jr, White EB: *The Elements of Style,* 3rd ed. New York, NY, Macmillan Publishing Co. Inc., 1979.

Sultz HA: *Grant Writing for Health Professionals.* Boston, Little, Brown, and Co., 1981.

Winer, BJ: *Statistical Principles in Experimental Design,* 2nd ed. New York, NY, McGraw-Hill, Inc., 1971.

Zeiger M: *Essentials of Writing Biomedical Research Papers.* New York, NY, McGraw-Hill, Inc., 1991.